TITLE: FITNESS GUIDE

INTRODUCTION

In today's fast-paced and sedentary lifestyle, maintaining optimal fitness has become more important than ever. As we juggle work, family, and other responsibilities, our physical and mental well-being often take a backseat. However, adopting a holistic approach to fitness can greatly enhance our quality of life and ensure we have the energy and vitality to tackle whatever challenges come our way.

The significance of fitness

Fitness goes beyond just having a fit physique; it encompasses physical, mental, and emotional well-being. Regular exercise and a balanced lifestyle not only improve our physical health but also boost our mood, enhance cognitive function, reduce stress, and increase our overall happiness. It is a powerful tool that empowers us to live our lives to the fullest.

Overview of the book's purpose

In this comprehensive guide, titled "The Fitness Guide," our aim is to provide readers with a step-by-step roadmap to achieving and maintaining optimal fitness. From understanding the components of fitness to setting goals, creating personalized workout and nutrition plans, and incorporating mindfulness and recovery techniques, this book will equip you with the knowledge and tools to embark on a transformative fitness journey. Whether you are a beginner or a fitness enthusiast looking to take your fitness to the next level, this book will serve as your trusted companion in achieving your goals.

By the end of this book, you will have a deeper understanding of fitness, the knowledge to create a personalized fitness plan, and the motivation to embrace fitness as a lifelong commitment. Get ready to embark on a transformative journey towards a healthier, fitter, and more vibrant version of yourself. The Fit Life awaits you!

THE IMPORTANCE OF FITNESS IN TODAY'S FAST-PACED, SEDENTARY LIFESTYLE.

In today's fast-paced and sedentary lifestyle, the importance of fitness cannot be overstated. As our lives become increasingly sedentary, with long hours spent sitting at desks or in front of screens, our physical activity levels have plummeted, leading to a myriad of health concerns. Incorporating fitness into our daily lives has become crucial for maintaining our well-being and vitality in the face of these challenges.

- ❖ **Sedentary lifestyle and its consequences:** The modern lifestyle, characterized by desk jobs, long commutes, and entertainment options that encourage prolonged sitting, has contributed to a decline in physical activity levels. This sedentary behavior has been linked to a host of health problems, including obesity, cardiovascular diseases, diabetes, musculoskeletal disorders, and even mental health issues such as anxiety and depression. The negative impacts of a sedentary lifestyle highlight the urgent need for regular exercise and physical activity.
- ❖ **Physical fitness and overall well-being:** Fitness plays a pivotal role in maintaining our physical health. Regular exercise strengthens our muscles, bones, and joints, improving our overall functional capacity and reducing the risk of chronic conditions. It enhances cardiovascular health, boosting heart function and lowering the risk of heart disease. Exercise also aids in weight management, as it helps burn calories and build lean muscle mass.
- ❖ **Beyond physical benefits:** Fitness extends beyond physical health. Engaging in regular exercise releases endorphins, neurotransmitters that promote feelings of happiness and well-being, thus improving

our mental and emotional state. Exercise has been proven to alleviate stress, reduce anxiety and depression, enhance cognitive function, and improve sleep quality. It provides a natural energy boost, combating fatigue and promoting productivity.

- ❖ **Quality of life:** By prioritizing fitness, we enhance our overall quality of life. Fitness promotes longevity, enabling us to enjoy our later years with vitality and independence. It increases our energy levels, enabling us to engage fully in our daily activities and pursuits. Additionally, a fit body and mind contribute to a positive body image and self-esteem, fostering confidence and self-assurance.
- ❖ **Nurturing a balanced lifestyle:** Integrating fitness into our lives encourages a balanced approach to overall well-being. It reminds us to prioritize self-care, carve out time for physical activity, and make conscious choices about nutrition and rest. A focus on fitness can inspire us to establish healthy habits and positive routines, leading to greater self-discipline and a more harmonious lifestyle.

THE SIGNIFICANCE OF ADOPTING A HOLISTIC APPROACH TO FITNESS ENCOMPASSING PHYSICAL, MENTAL, AND EMOTIONAL WELL-BEING

When it comes to achieving optimal fitness, taking a holistic approach that encompasses physical, mental, and emotional well-being is of utmost significance. A narrow focus on physical fitness alone overlooks the interconnectedness of these dimensions and fails to address the full spectrum of our well-being. By adopting a holistic approach, we unlock the true potential of our fitness journey and cultivate a sustainable, balanced, and fulfilling lifestyle.

- ❖ **Physical well-being:** Physical fitness is the foundation of our overall well-being. Engaging in regular exercise and maintaining a healthy lifestyle strengthens our cardiovascular system, builds muscle strength, improves flexibility, and promotes a healthy body composition. A strong physical foundation not only enhances our functional abilities but also protects us against illness and disease, increases our energy levels, and promotes longevity.

- ❖ **Mental well-being:** The mind-body connection is undeniable, and mental well-being is a vital component of holistic fitness. Regular exercise has been proven to alleviate stress, reduce anxiety and depression, boost mood, and enhance cognitive function. Physical activity stimulates the release of endorphins, neurotransmitters that promote feelings of happiness and well-being. By prioritizing mental well-being, we foster mental clarity, resilience, and emotional balance, enabling us to navigate life's challenges with greater ease.

- ❖ **Emotional well-being:** Emotions play a significant role in our overall health and fitness journey. Adopting a holistic approach means recognizing and nurturing our emotional well-being. Engaging in physical activity provides an outlet for stress, anger, and other intense emotions. It cultivates self-awareness, allowing us to process and manage our emotions more effectively. By integrating practices such as mindfulness and self-reflection, we develop emotional intelligence, resilience, and a sense of inner peace.

- ❖ **Balance and synergy:** Taking a holistic approach to fitness recognizes the synergy between physical, mental, and emotional well-being. When we focus solely on physical fitness, neglecting our mental and emotional health, imbalances can arise, leading to burnout, low motivation, and unsustainable habits. By nurturing all aspects of our well-being, we create a harmonious and sustainable fitness journey. The balance between physical, mental, and emotional health creates a positive feedback loop, where improvements in one area support growth in the others.

- ❖ **Long-term sustainability:** A holistic approach to fitness fosters long-term sustainability. It acknowledges that fitness is not a destination but a lifelong journey. By considering our physical, mental, and emotional well-being, we create a foundation for lasting habits and lifestyle changes. This approach allows us to adapt to the evolving demands of life, adjust our routines when necessary, and maintain a consistent commitment to our fitness goals.

Conclusion:By nurturing and balancing all aspects of our well-being, we create a sustainable and fulfilling lifestyle that promotes optimal fitness, resilience, and overall wellness. Remember, true fitness is achieved when we strive for harmony within ourselves, acknowledging the interconnectedness of our physical, mental, and emotional selves.

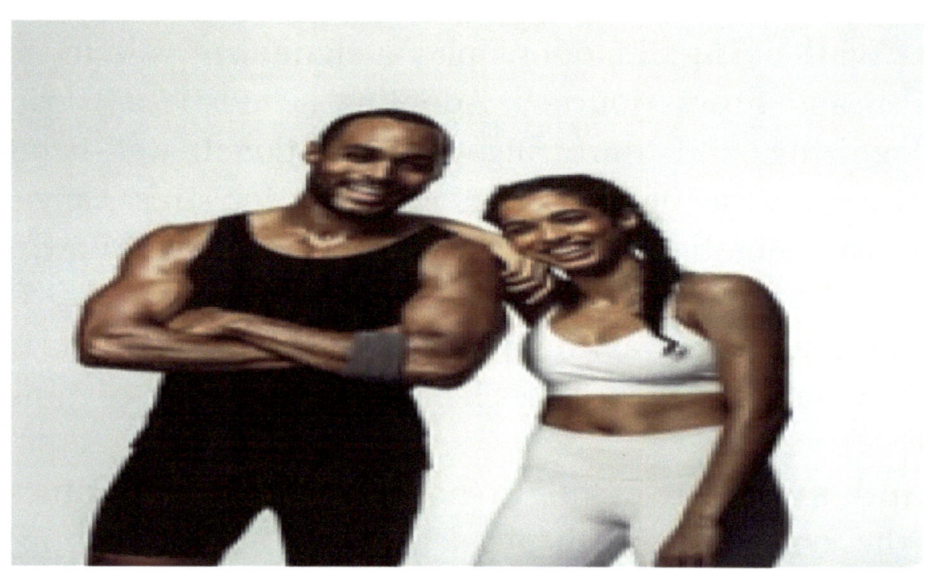

In this book "A Comprehensive Fitness Guide to Achieving Optimal Fitness and Well-being," our purpose is to equip readers with a practical and step-by-step roadmap to achieving and maintaining optimal fitness. Whether you are a beginner starting your fitness journey or a fitness enthusiast looking to take your fitness to the next level, this book will serve as your trusted companion in achieving your goals.

❖ **Understanding fitness:** We begin by providing a clear definition of fitness and exploring its various components, including cardiovascular endurance, muscular strength and endurance, flexibility, and body composition. By understanding the different facets of fitness, readers can gain a holistic perspective and set comprehensive goals.

- ❖ **Nutrition for fitness:** Recognizing the significance of nutrition in achieving optimal fitness, we provide a thorough exploration of the role of macronutrients (carbohydrates, proteins, and fats) and micronutrients in fueling the body for exercise and supporting overall health. Readers will learn strategies for balanced and healthy eating, portion control, and mindful eating practices, debunking common nutritional myths along the way.
- ❖ **Strength training:** We dive into the realm of strength training, highlighting its benefits for overall fitness. Readers will learn about different types of strength training exercises, such as bodyweight exercises, free weights, and machines. Proper form and technique will be emphasized, along with guidance on developing a well-rounded strength training program targeting major muscle groups.
- ❖ **Cardiovascular exercise:** Recognizing the importance of cardiovascular exercise for heart health and endurance, we explore various cardio activities such as running, cycling, swimming, and high-intensity interval training (HIIT). Readers will discover how to design effective cardio workout routines based on their fitness level and goals, incorporating interval training and progressive overload for optimal results.
- ❖ **Flexibility and mobility:** We emphasize the significance of flexibility and mobility in preventing injuries and maintaining functional movement. Readers will learn stretching techniques such as static, dynamic, and proprioceptive neuromuscular facilitation (PNF) stretching. The book will also provide guidance on incorporating mobility exercises and foam rolling into the fitness routine, along with warm-up and cool-down routines.
- ❖ **Mind-body connection:** Acknowledging the connection between mental well-being and physical fitness, we explore the benefits of mindfulness, meditation, and stress management techniques. Readers will discover the integration of yoga and Pilates for improved

flexibility, strength, and mental clarity. Strategies for maintaining motivation, dealing with setbacks, and fostering a positive mindset will also be shared.

- ❖ **Recovery and injury prevention:** Recognizing the importance of recovery for optimal fitness gains, we delve into various recovery techniques, including sleep, nutrition, and active rest. Readers will learn about injury prevention through proper form and technique, as well as strategies for rehabilitation and injury management. We also address the risks of overtraining and burnout, providing strategies for avoiding them.

- ❖ **Tracking progress and adjusting the plan:** We emphasize the importance of monitoring and evaluating fitness progress through tracking measurements, strength gains, and endurance improvements. Readers will learn how to modify their fitness plan to accommodate changing goals and circumstances, seek professional guidance and support, and address plateaus by adapting their routine for continued progress.

Conclusion: By the end of this book, you will have gained a deeper understanding of fitness, the tools to set effective goals, the knowledge to create a personalized fitness plan, and the motivation to embrace fitness as a lifelong commitment. "The Fit Life"

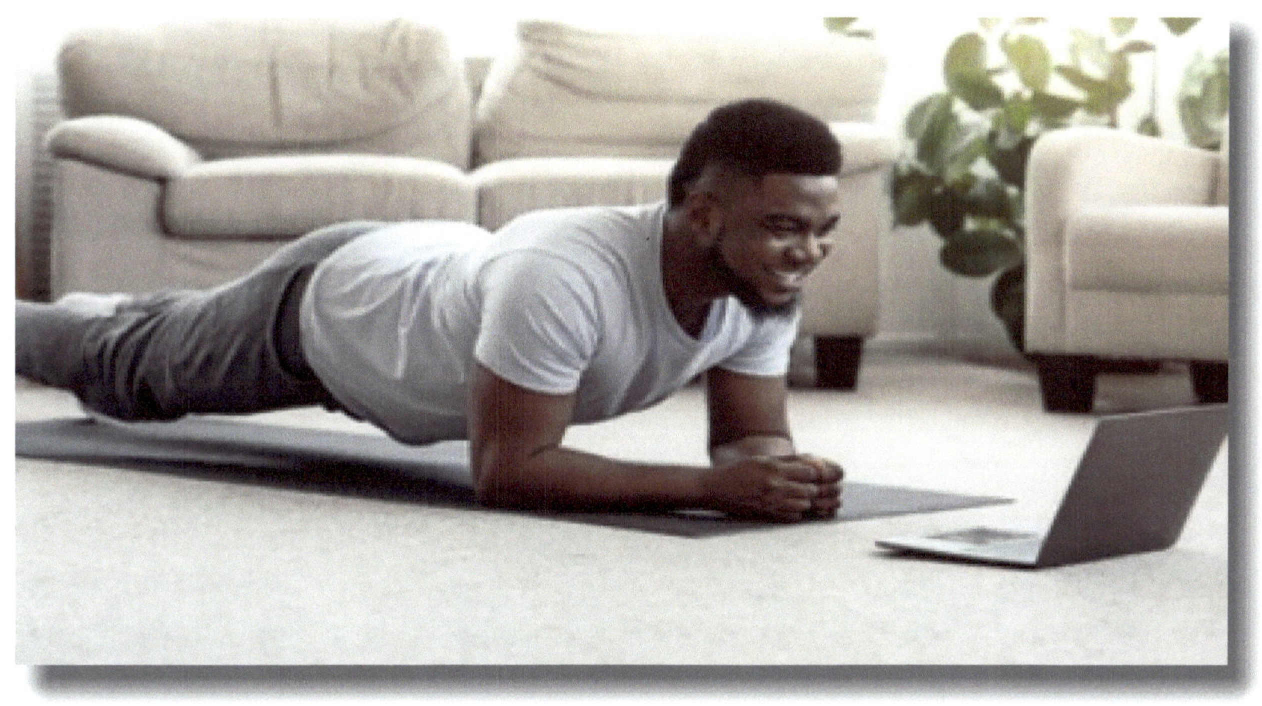

CHAPTER ONE: UNDERSTANDING FITNESS

DEFINITION OF FITNESS AND ITS COMPONENTS

Fitness refers to the overall state of being physically and mentally healthy, characterized by the ability to perform daily activities with vigor, efficiency, and resilience. It encompasses various components that contribute to one's physical well-being and overall quality of life.

Cardiovascular endurance, also known as cardiorespiratory endurance or aerobic fitness, is the ability of the heart, lungs, and circulatory system to efficiently deliver oxygen and nutrients to the muscles during sustained physical activity. It reflects the body's capacity to sustain prolonged exercise and engage in activities that elevate the heart rate, such as running, swimming, cycling, or brisk walking.

Muscular strength refers to the maximal force a muscle or group of muscles can generate against resistance. It is essential for activities that require power and explosiveness, such as weightlifting or sprinting.

Muscular endurance, on the other hand, refers to the ability of a muscle or muscle group to sustain repeated contractions over an extended period. It is crucial for activities that involve repetitive movements, like long-distance running or cycling.

Flexibility refers to the range of motion around a joint or series of joints. It is determined by the elasticity and length of muscles, tendons, ligaments, and other connective tissues. Maintaining good flexibility enhances physical performance, reduces the risk of injuries, and enables efficient movement patterns. Activities such as stretching, yoga, and Pilates are commonly used to improve flexibility.

Body composition refers to the proportion of different tissues that make up a person's total body weight. It includes fat mass, lean mass (muscle, bones, organs), and other components. Achieving a healthy body composition involves maintaining an appropriate balance between fat mass and lean mass. Regular exercise, combined with a nutritious diet, plays a vital role in achieving and maintaining a healthy body composition.

These components of fitness are interconnected, and a well-rounded fitness program should address all of them. By improving cardiovascular endurance, muscular strength and endurance, flexibility, and body composition, individuals can enhance their overall fitness and improve their overall health and well-being.

EXPLORING THE BENEFITS OF REGULAR EXERCISE AND PHYSICAL ACTIVITY

Regular exercise and physical activity offer a wide range of benefits that positively impact various aspects of our lives. Here are some key benefits of incorporating regular exercise into our routines:

- ❖ **Improved Physical Health:** Engaging in regular exercise promotes cardiovascular health by strengthening the heart, improving circulation, and reducing the risk of cardiovascular diseases such as heart disease and stroke. It also helps maintain a healthy body weight, lowers blood pressure, improves cholesterol levels, and enhances overall metabolic function. Regular physical activity is associated with a decreased risk of chronic conditions such as obesity, type 2 diabetes, certain types of cancer, and osteoporosis.

- ❖ **Enhanced Mental Health and Well-being:** Exercise has a profound impact on mental health by boosting mood and reducing symptoms of depression, anxiety, and stress. Physical activity stimulates the release of endorphins, which are natural mood-enhancing chemicals in the brain. Regular exercise also improves cognitive function, memory, and attention, promoting mental sharpness and reducing the risk of age-related cognitive decline. It can provide a sense of accomplishment, self-confidence, and increased self-esteem.

- ❖ **Weight Management:** Regular exercise, combined with a balanced diet, plays a crucial role in maintaining a healthy body weight. It helps burn calories, build muscle mass, and increase metabolism, contributing to weight loss or weight maintenance. Exercise also helps prevent weight regain after weight loss, making it an essential component of long-term weight management.

- ❖ **Increased Energy and Stamina:** Engaging in regular physical activity enhances energy levels and reduces fatigue. It improves muscular strength, endurance, and overall stamina, enabling individuals to perform daily tasks with greater ease and efficiency. Regular exercise also improves sleep quality, promoting better rest and rejuvenation.

- ❖ **Stronger Muscles, Bones, and Joints:** Exercise that includes resistance training, such as weightlifting or bodyweight exercises, helps build and strengthen muscles. This not only improves physical performance but also supports the health and stability of joints. Weight-bearing exercises, including walking or jogging, help maintain bone density and reduce the risk of osteoporosis, especially in older adults.

- ❖ **Improved Flexibility and Balance**: Incorporating flexibility exercises, such as stretching or yoga, into a fitness routine enhances joint flexibility, range of motion, and overall mobility. This can improve posture, reduce the risk of injuries, and enhance balance, particularly in older adults.

- ❖ **Longevity and Quality of Life:** Regular exercise has been linked to increased longevity and a better quality of life. It reduces the risk of premature death and age-related health issues, allowing individuals to maintain independence, vitality, and an active lifestyle as they age.
- ❖ **Social and Emotional Benefits:** Participating in group fitness classes, team sports, or exercising with friends and family can provide social connections, support, and motivation. Regular exercise can also be a positive outlet for managing stress, enhancing self-confidence, and improving overall emotional well-being.

In summary, regular exercise and physical activity offer a multitude of benefits for physical health, mental well-being, weight management, energy levels, muscle and bone strength, flexibility, balance, longevity, and social connections. By making exercise a consistent part of our lives, we can experience these positive effects and lead healthier, happier lives.

DEBUNKING COMMON FITNESS MYTHS AND MISCONCEPTIONS

- ❖ **Myth 1:** Spot reduction of fat is possible. Debunking: Targeting specific areas of the body for fat loss, such as doing endless crunches to get rid of belly fat, is a common misconception. In reality, fat loss occurs throughout the body as a whole. To reduce body fat in a particular area, it's necessary to engage in overall fat loss through a combination of regular exercise, a balanced diet, and maintaining a calorie deficit.
- ❖ **Myth 2:** Lifting weights will make women bulky. Debunking: This is a prevalent myth that discourages many women from strength training. In reality, women have lower testosterone levels compared to men, which limits their muscle-building potential. Strength training actually helps women build lean muscle, improve muscle tone, increase metabolism, and enhance overall body composition. It promotes a fit and toned appearance rather than bulkiness.

- ❖ **Myth 3:** Cardio is the best way to lose weight. Debunking: While cardiovascular exercise contributes to calorie burning, weight loss is most effective when combined with a well-rounded fitness routine that includes both cardiovascular exercise and strength training. Strength training helps build muscle, which increases metabolism and leads to more efficient fat burning even at rest. A combination of both cardio and strength training is the ideal approach for weight loss and overall fitness.
- ❖ **Myth 4:** No pain, no gain. Debunking: Pushing through extreme pain or discomfort during exercise is not necessary and can lead to injury. While some muscle soreness is normal when starting a new exercise program or increasing intensity, it's essential to listen to your body and distinguish between muscle fatigue and sharp pain. Progressing gradually, using proper form, and allowing adequate rest and recovery are vital for long-term progress and injury prevention.
- ❖ **Myth 5:** You can exercise away a bad diet. Debunking: Nutrition and exercise go hand in hand when it comes to achieving fitness goals. While exercise plays a crucial role in overall health, it cannot compensate for a consistently poor diet. To optimize results, it's important to adopt a balanced, nutrient-rich diet that supports your fitness goals. A combination of healthy eating and regular exercise is key to achieving and maintaining optimal fitness.
- ❖ **Myth 6:** More exercise is always better. Debunking: While exercise is beneficial, more is not always better. Overtraining can lead to fatigue, increased risk of injury, hormonal imbalances, and impaired immune function. It's important to find a balance between challenging workouts and allowing adequate time for rest and recovery. Recovery days, proper sleep, and listening to your body's signals are crucial for long-term progress and overall well-being.
- ❖ **Myth 7:** You need expensive equipment or a gym membership to get fit. Debunking: Fitness can be achieved without expensive equipment or a gym membership. There are numerous bodyweight exercises, such as push-ups, squats, and lunges, that can be done anywhere. Walking, jogging, or running outdoors is a cost-effective way to engage in cardiovascular exercise. Additionally, there are plenty of

online resources, fitness apps, and home workout programs that offer guidance and support without the need for expensive equipment or gym access.

By dispelling these common fitness myths and misconceptions, individuals can make informed decisions, set realistic expectations, and adopt effective strategies to achieve their fitness goals. It's important to rely on evidence-based information, consult professionals when needed, and embrace a balanced and sustainable approach to fitness.

ASSESSING INDIVIDUAL FITNESS LEVELS: FITNESS TESTS AND MEASUREMENTS.

Assessing individual fitness levels is crucial to understanding current fitness status, identifying areas for improvement, and tracking progress over time. Here are some commonly used fitness tests and measurements:

- ❖ **Body Composition Analysis:** This test assesses the proportion of fat, muscle, and other tissues in the body. It can be done using various methods, such as skinfold calipers, bioelectrical impedance analysis (BIA), or dual-energy X-ray absorptiometry (DXA). Body mass index (BMI) is another measurement that estimates body fat based on height and weight, although it has limitations and may not accurately reflect individual body composition.
- ❖ **Cardiovascular Fitness Test:** The most popular test for cardiovascular fitness is the maximal oxygen consumption (VO2 max) test. It measures the body's ability to utilize oxygen during intense exercise. This test is often conducted on a treadmill or stationary bike while monitoring heart rate, oxygen consumption, and ventilation. Other simpler alternatives include the 1-mile walk/run test or the 3-minute step test.
- ❖ **Muscular Strength and Endurance Tests:** These tests evaluate the strength and endurance of specific muscle groups. Common tests include the one-repetition maximum (1RM) test, which determines the maximum weight an individual can lift for a single repetition.

Push-up and sit-up tests assess upper body and core strength and endurance, while the plank test measures core stability.

- ❖ **Flexibility Tests:** Flexibility assessments involve measuring the range of motion around specific joints or muscle groups. Tests such as the sit-and-reach test or shoulder flexibility test can provide an indication of overall flexibility and highlight areas that require improvement.
- ❖ **Balance and Stability Tests:** Balance assessments evaluate an individual's ability to maintain equilibrium. The single-leg balance test, the Romberg test, or the Y balance test are examples of tests that assess balance and stability.
- ❖ **Agility and Speed Tests:** Agility and speed tests measure an individual's ability to change direction quickly, accelerate, and reach maximal velocity. The 40-yard dash, shuttle run, or T-test are commonly used tests to assess agility and speed.
- ❖ **Functional Movement Assessments:** Functional movement assessments evaluate movement patterns and identify any imbalances, weaknesses, or limitations that may increase the risk of injury. The Functional Movement Screen (FMS) is a widely used test that assesses seven fundamental movement patterns.

It's important to note that fitness tests and measurements should be conducted by qualified professionals to ensure accuracy and safety. The results of these assessments provide valuable information that can guide the development of personalized fitness programs, set specific goals, and track progress over time. Additionally, consulting with a healthcare professional or fitness expert can help interpret the results and create a plan to improve areas of weakness and enhance overall fitness.

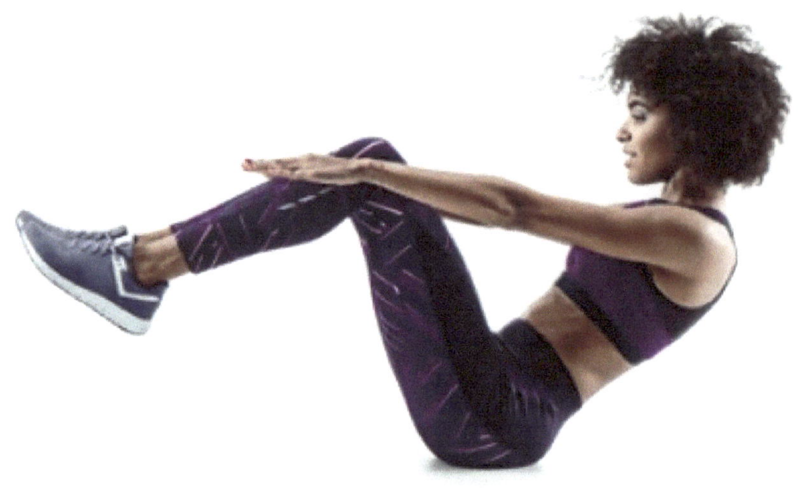

CHAPTER TWO: SETTING GOALS AND CREATING A PLAN

IDENTIFYING PERSONAL FITNESS GOALS

When identifying personal fitness goals, it's important to consider individual preferences, current fitness level, and desired outcomes. Here are some common fitness goals:

- ❖ **Weight Loss:** Many individuals aim to lose weight for health or aesthetic reasons. Weight loss goals can be achieved through a combination of regular exercise, a balanced and calorie-controlled diet, and a sustainable approach to lifestyle changes.
- ❖ **Muscle Gain and Strength:** Some individuals focus on building muscle mass and increasing overall strength. This goal typically involves resistance training exercises that target specific muscle groups, progressive overload (gradually increasing the weight or intensity of exercises), and consuming adequate protein to support muscle growth.
- ❖ **Increased Endurance:** Endurance goals revolve around improving cardiovascular fitness, stamina, and the ability to sustain physical activity for extended periods. Aerobic exercises like running, cycling,

swimming, or participating in endurance events like marathons or triathlons can help improve endurance.

- ❖ **Flexibility and Mobility:** Enhancing flexibility and mobility is a common goal for individuals looking to improve range of motion, prevent injuries, and promote overall physical well-being. Stretching exercises, yoga, Pilates, and mobility drills can help achieve greater flexibility and improved movement patterns.
- ❖ **Functional Fitness:** Functional fitness goals focus on improving physical abilities required for daily activities or specific sports or occupations. This may involve exercises that mimic real-life movements, balance and stability training, and core strength development.
- ❖ **Stress Reduction and Mental Well-being:** Fitness goals aren't limited to physical outcomes. Many people prioritize exercise for its mental and emotional benefits, aiming to reduce stress, boost mood, improve sleep, and enhance overall mental well-being. Activities like yoga, meditation, or mindfulness practices can complement physical exercise in achieving these goals.
- ❖ **Sports-specific Performance:** Athletes or individuals engaged in specific sports may have goals centered around improving performance in their chosen activity. These goals may include increasing speed, agility, power, or sport-specific skills through targeted training programs.

Remember, goals should be specific, measurable, achievable, relevant, and time-bound (SMART). It's important to set realistic goals that align with personal capabilities and lifestyle factors. Consulting with a fitness professional or healthcare provider can help assess individual needs and create a personalized plan to achieve desired fitness goals. Regular progress assessments and modifications to the fitness program may be necessary to stay motivated and on track.

CREATING A PERSONALIZED FITNESS PLAN: SELECTING SUITABLE EXERCISES AND ACTIVITIES.

Creating a personalized fitness plan involves selecting exercises and activities that align with your goals, preferences, fitness level, and available resources. Here's a step-by-step process to help you create a tailored fitness plan:

- ❖ **Identify Your Goals:** Determine what you want to achieve through your fitness plan. Is it weight loss, muscle gain, increased endurance, improved flexibility, or a combination of these? Clearly defining your goals will help guide your exercise selection.
- ❖ **Assess Your Current Fitness Level:** Evaluate your current fitness level to determine your starting point. Consider factors such as cardiovascular fitness, muscular strength, flexibility, and overall mobility. This assessment will help you gauge your capabilities and set realistic expectations for your fitness plan.
- ❖ **Consider Your Preferences:** Choose exercises and activities that you enjoy and are likely to stick with in the long term. Consider activities such as running, cycling, swimming, dancing, martial arts, weightlifting, group fitness classes, yoga, or sports. By selecting activities, you genuinely enjoy, you'll be more motivated to engage in them consistently.
- ❖ **Determine Exercise Types:** A well-rounded fitness plan includes a combination of cardiovascular exercise, strength training, flexibility training, and functional movements. Cardiovascular exercises, such as jogging, cycling, or dancing, improve heart health and endurance. Strength training exercises, like weightlifting or bodyweight exercises, build muscle strength and increase metabolism. Flexibility exercises, such as stretching or yoga, enhance mobility and prevent injuries. Functional movements involve exercises that mimic real-life activities and improve overall functionality.
- ❖ **Choose Frequency and Duration: Decide** how many days per week you can commit to your fitness plan and allocate appropriate durations for each session. The American College of Sports Medicine

recommends at least 150 minutes of moderate-intensity aerobic exercise or 75 minutes of vigorous-intensity aerobic exercise per week, along with two or more days of strength training.

- ❖ **Plan Progression:** Gradually increase the intensity, duration, or difficulty of your workouts over time. This progression is essential to continually challenge your body and avoid plateauing. Start with manageable workout routines and gradually increase the intensity, frequency, or duration as your fitness level improves.
- ❖ **Incorporate Rest and Recovery:** Allow time for rest and recovery between workouts. Adequate rest is crucial for muscle repair and growth, injury prevention, and overall well-being. Plan rest days or incorporate lighter activities, such as stretching or gentle yoga, on these days.
- ❖ **Consider Safety and Injury Prevention:** Prioritize proper form and technique when performing exercises to prevent injuries. If you're new to certain activities, consider seeking guidance from fitness professionals or trainers to ensure correct form and reduce the risk of injury.
- ❖ **Track Your Progress:** Keep a record of your workouts, including exercises, sets, reps, and weights. Regularly reassess your goals and track your progress to stay motivated and make necessary adjustments to your fitness plan.
- ❖ **Stay Flexible:** Be open to modifying your fitness plan as needed. Life circumstances, interests, and fitness goals may change over time. It's essential to remain flexible and adapt your plan accordingly to ensure its long-term sustainability.

Remember, consulting with a healthcare professional or certified fitness expert can provide personalized guidance and help tailor a fitness plan specific to your needs and limitations. They can assist with exercise selection, form correction, and provide additional support along your fitness journey.

Periodization is a training concept that involves organizing workouts into distinct phases or periods to optimize long-term progress and prevent plateaus. It provides a systematic approach to training that takes into account various factors, such as goals, fitness level, recovery, and specific time frames. The main idea behind periodization is to introduce planned variations in training variables to stimulate continuous adaptation and avoid stagnation.

Here are the key components of periodization:

- ❖ **Phases:** Periodization typically consists of three main phases: macrocycle, mesocycle, and microcycle.
- ❖ **Macrocycle:** This is the long-term plan that encompasses your overall training timeline, often spanning several months or even a year. It includes multiple mesocycles and is designed to achieve specific goals.
- ❖ **Mesocycle:** This phase breaks down the macrocycle into more manageable segments, typically lasting a few weeks to a few months. Each mesocycle focuses on a specific aspect of fitness, such as building strength, improving endurance, or enhancing power.
- ❖ **Microcycle:** The microcycle represents the smallest training unit within the mesocycle, typically spanning one week. It outlines the daily or weekly training sessions and their specific objectives.
- ❖ **Training Variables:** Periodization involves manipulating various training variables throughout the different phases to promote adaptation and avoid plateaus. These variables include intensity, volume, frequency, and exercise selection.
- ❖ **Intensity:** Refers to the level of effort or resistance applied during a workout. It can be adjusted by manipulating weights, speeds, or percentages of maximum effort.
- ❖ **Volume:** Represents the total amount of work performed in a training session or over a specific time period. It can be measured by the number of sets, reps, or duration of training sessions.

- ❖ **Frequency:** Refers to how often training sessions occur. It can be adjusted by varying the number of workouts per week.
- ❖ **Exercise Selection:** Involves choosing specific exercises that target the desired training goals and the corresponding muscle groups.
- ❖ **Periodization Models:** Different periodization models exist, each with its own unique structure. Common models include linear periodization, undulating periodization, and conjugate periodization. These models vary in the way they manipulate training variables and progress over time.
- ❖ **Adaptation and Recovery:** Periodization incorporates planned periods of recovery and adaptation to prevent overtraining and allow the body to adapt to the training stimulus. These recovery periods may involve reducing training volume, intensity, or frequency to allow for adequate rest and recuperation.

Benefits of Periodization:

- ❖ **Progressive Overload:** Periodization ensures that the training stimulus progressively increases over time, allowing for continued adaptation and improvement.
- ❖ **Avoiding Plateaus:** By systematically varying training variables, periodization helps prevent plateaus and keeps the body challenged. It introduces new exercises, intensity levels, or training methods to stimulate further progress.
- ❖ **Injury Prevention:** Periodization allows for planned recovery periods, reducing the risk of overuse injuries. It also helps balance the workload on different muscle groups and avoids excessive stress on the body.
- ❖ **Goal-Specific Training:** Periodization allows for targeted training phases that address specific fitness goals. Whether it's building strength, increasing endurance, or improving power, periodization can tailor the training program to align with specific objectives.
- ❖ **Long-Term Planning:** By structuring training into distinct phases, periodization promotes a long-term approach to fitness. It helps individuals track progress, set realistic expectations, and maintain motivation over an extended period.

Periodization is a valuable tool for athletes, fitness enthusiasts, and individuals seeking long-term progress and performance enhancement. It provides a structured framework to optimize training outcomes, prevent plateaus, and achieve sustainable results. Working with a qualified fitness professional or coach can help tailor a periodized training plan

CHAPTER THREE: NUTRITION FOR FITNESS

UNDERSTANDING THE ROLE OF NUTRITION IN ACHIEVING FITNESS GOALS

Nutrition plays a vital role in achieving fitness goals as it provides the body with the necessary fuel, nutrients, and building blocks for optimal performance, recovery, and overall health. Here are some key aspects of nutrition in relation to fitness:

- ❖ **Energy Balance:** Achieving and maintaining a healthy body weight is often a key aspect of fitness goals. Energy balance is the relationship between the calories consumed through food and the calories expended through physical activity. To lose weight, a calorie deficit is needed, while a calorie surplus is required for muscle gain. Balancing energy intake with expenditure is crucial for achieving body composition goals.
- ❖ **Macronutrients:** Macronutrients are the three main nutrients required in relatively large amounts: carbohydrates, proteins, and fats.

  Carbohydrates provide energy for exercise and replenish glycogen stores in muscles. They are particularly important for high-intensity activities and endurance exercises. Focus on consuming complex carbohydrates, such as whole grains, fruits, vegetables, and legumes.

  Proteins are essential for repairing and building muscle tissue, supporting immune function, and various physiological processes. Adequate protein intake is crucial for muscle growth and recovery. Sources of protein include lean meats, poultry, fish, dairy products, legumes, nuts, and seeds.

  Fats provide energy, support hormone production, and aid in nutrient absorption. Opt for healthy fats, such as those found in avocados, nuts, seeds, olive oil, and fatty fish like salmon.
- ❖ **Micronutrients:** Micronutrients include vitamins and minerals, which are essential for various physiological functions, including energy metabolism, bone health, immune function, and muscle contraction. Consuming a variety of fruits, vegetables, whole grains,

lean proteins, and dairy products can help ensure an adequate intake of micronutrients.

- ❖ **Hydration:** Proper hydration is crucial for optimal physical performance. Water is involved in nearly all bodily processes and is especially important for temperature regulation, joint lubrication, nutrient transport, and waste removal. Aim to drink water consistently throughout the day and increase intake during exercise or in hot weather.
- ❖ **Timing of Meals and Snacks:** Pay attention to the timing of meals and snacks to optimize energy levels and recovery. Consuming a balanced meal containing carbohydrates, protein, and healthy fats about 2-3 hours before exercise can provide sustained energy. Additionally, refueling with a combination of carbohydrates and protein within 30 minutes to 2 hours after exercise supports muscle recovery.
- ❖ **Individualized Approach:** Each person's nutritional needs may vary based on factors such as age, sex, weight, activity level, and specific fitness goals. Consulting with a registered dietitian or nutritionist can help develop an individualized nutrition plan that aligns with your goals and optimizes performance.

It's important to note that nutrition alone cannot guarantee fitness goals. It should be combined with regular exercise, proper rest and recovery, and a holistic lifestyle approach. Adopting a balanced and sustainable approach to nutrition will not only support your fitness goals but also promote overall well-being and long-term health.

THE BASICS OF MACRONUTRIENTS (CARBOHYDRATES, PROTEINS, AND FATS) AND THEIR IMPORTANCE.

Macronutrients are the three main nutrients that the body requires in larger quantities to provide energy, support bodily functions, and promote overall health. Understanding the basics of macronutrients, including carbohydrates, proteins, and fats, is crucial for maintaining a balanced and nutritious diet. Here's an overview of each macronutrient and its importance:

Carbohydrates:

Role: Carbohydrates are the body's primary source of energy. They provide fuel for physical activity, brain function, and various physiological processes.

Types: Carbohydrates can be categorized into two main types: simple carbohydrates and complex carbohydrates.

- ❖ Simple carbohydrates, also known as sugars, are found in foods such as fruits, vegetables, and refined sugars (e.g., table sugar, honey, syrups). They are quickly digested and provide a rapid source of energy.
- ❖ Complex carbohydrates, also known as starches, are found in foods such as whole grains, legumes, and starchy vegetables. They are composed of longer chains of sugar molecules and provide sustained energy due to their slower digestion and release of glucose into the bloodstream.

Importance: Carbohydrates play a vital role in high-intensity exercise and endurance activities. They replenish glycogen stores in muscles, support brain function, and spare protein for other important functions.

Proteins:

Role: Proteins are essential for building, repairing, and maintaining tissues in the body. They are composed of amino acids, which are the building blocks of proteins. Proteins are involved in various functions, including muscle development, immune function, enzyme production, and hormone regulation.

Sources: Proteins are found in both animal and plant-based foods. Animal sources include meat, poultry, fish, eggs, and dairy products. Plant-based sources include legumes (beans, lentils), tofu, tempeh, seitan, nuts, seeds, and certain grains (quinoa, amaranth).

Importance: Protein is crucial for muscle growth, repair, and recovery. It plays a significant role in supporting strength and endurance during exercise. Adequate protein intake is essential for individuals looking to build and maintain lean muscle mass, especially those engaged in strength training or intense physical activity.

Fats:

Role: Fats serve as an essential energy source, provide insulation and protection to organs, support hormone production, aid in nutrient absorption (fat-soluble vitamins), and contribute to cell structure and function.

Types: Fats can be categorized into saturated fats, unsaturated fats (monounsaturated and polyunsaturated fats), and trans fats.

- ❖ Saturated fats are primarily found in animal-based foods (meat, butter, full-fat dairy products) and some plant-based sources (coconut oil, palm oil). High intake of saturated fats may increase the risk of cardiovascular diseases.
- ❖ Unsaturated fats are considered healthier fats and can be found in foods such as avocados, nuts, seeds, olive oil, and fatty fish (salmon, mackerel). They are beneficial for heart health when consumed in moderation.
- ❖ Trans fats are artificial fats created through a process called hydrogenation and are commonly found in processed foods, fried foods, and commercially baked goods. Trans fats should be limited or avoided due to their negative impact on heart health.

Importance: Fats help with the absorption of fat-soluble vitamins (A, D, E, and K) and provide a concentrated source of energy. They also play a role in maintaining healthy cell membranes, supporting brain function, and providing insulation and protection to organs.

It's important to note that a well-balanced diet should include all three macronutrients in appropriate proportions. The specific macronutrient

STRATEGIES FOR BALANCED AND HEALTHY EATING, INCLUDING PORTION CONTROL AND MINDFUL EATING.

Maintaining a balanced and healthy eating pattern is crucial for overall well-being, supporting fitness goals, and promoting optimal health. Here are some strategies for achieving balanced and healthy eating:

Portion Control:

- ❖ **Be mindful of portion sizes:** Understanding appropriate portion sizes can help prevent overeating. Use visual cues, such as using your hand or familiar objects, to estimate portion sizes for different food groups.
- ❖ **Read food labels:** Pay attention to serving sizes listed on food labels to ensure you're consuming appropriate portions.
- ❖ **Use smaller plates and bowls:** Opting for smaller plates and bowls can create an illusion of a fuller plate, helping to control portion sizes.

Mindful Eating:

- ❖ **Slow down and savor your meals:** Take your time to fully experience and enjoy the flavors, textures, and aromas of your food. Eating slowly can help you recognize satiety cues and prevent overeating.
- ❖ **Pay attention to hunger and fullness cues:** Eat when you're hungry and stop when you're comfortably full. Tune in to your body's signals and avoid eating out of boredom, stress, or emotions.
- ❖ **Minimize distractions:** Avoid eating in front of screens or while engaged in other activities. Focus on your meal, allowing yourself to fully engage with the eating experience.

❖ **Practice gratitude:** Take a moment before your meal to express gratitude for the food on your plate and the nourishment it provides.

Include a Variety of Foods:

❖ **Eat a rainbow of fruits and vegetables:** Aim to include a wide variety of colorful fruits and vegetables in your diet. They provide essential vitamins, minerals, and antioxidants.

❖ **Choose whole grains:** Opt for whole grains such as quinoa, brown rice, whole wheat bread, and oats instead of refined grains. Whole grains provide fiber and important nutrients.

❖ **Include lean proteins:** Incorporate lean sources of protein, such as poultry, fish, beans, lentils, tofu, and Greek yogurt, to support muscle growth and repair.

❖ **Healthy fats:** Include sources of healthy fats, such as avocados, nuts, seeds, and olive oil, in moderation to support overall health and satiety.

Plan and Prepare Meals:

❖ **Plan ahead:** Take time to plan your meals and snacks for the week. This helps you make healthier choices, avoid impulsive decisions, and stay on track with your nutrition goals.

❖ **Prepare meals at home:** Cooking meals at home allows you to have more control over the ingredients and portion sizes. Experiment with new recipes and cooking techniques to make healthy eating enjoyable.

❖ **Batch cook and meal prep:** Consider preparing larger quantities of food and portioning them out for future meals. This can save time and make it easier to choose healthy options when you're busy or on the go.

Stay Hydrated:

❖ **Drink water throughout the day:** Aim to drink an adequate amount of water to stay hydrated. Water is essential for digestion, nutrient absorption, temperature regulation, and overall well-being.

- ❖ **Limit sugary beverages:** Minimize or avoid sugary drinks such as soda, fruit juices, energy drinks, and sweetened coffee or tea. Opt for water, herbal tea, or infused water for hydration.

Remember, balanced and healthy eating is not about strict rules or deprivation. It's about nourishing your body with a variety of nutrient-dense foods, practicing portion control, and cultivating a positive relationship with food. Seek guidance from a registered dietitian or nutritionist for personalized advice and support in developing a sustainable and enjoyable eating pattern.

ADDRESSING COMMON NUTRITIONAL CHALLENGES AND MISCONCEPTIONS

When it comes to nutrition, there are several common challenges and misconceptions that can hinder progress towards optimal health and fitness goals. Addressing these challenges and misconceptions is important for promoting accurate and evidence-based information. Here are some common nutritional challenges and misconceptions:

Restrictive Diets:

- ❖ **Challenge:** Following overly restrictive diets or fad diets that eliminate entire food groups or severely restrict calorie intake can lead to nutrient deficiencies, unsustainable eating habits, and negative effects on metabolism.
- ❖ **Addressing the misconception:** Emphasize the importance of a balanced and varied diet that includes all major food groups. Encourage individuals to focus on nourishing their bodies with whole, minimally processed foods rather than relying on quick fixes or extreme measures.

Micronutrient Deficiencies:

- ❖ **Challenge:** Inadequate intake of essential vitamins and minerals can lead to deficiencies, impacting overall health and performance.
- ❖ **Addressing the misconception:** Educate individuals about the importance of consuming a wide variety of nutrient-dense foods to

ensure an adequate intake of micronutrients. Emphasize the benefits of incorporating fruits, vegetables, whole grains, lean proteins, and healthy fats into daily meals and snacks.

Misunderstanding of Carbohydrates:

* ❖ **Challenge:** Carbohydrates often receive negative attention, leading to misconceptions that they are inherently unhealthy or promote weight gain.
* ❖ **Addressing the misconception:** Explain the role of carbohydrates as the body's primary source of energy and the importance of consuming complex carbohydrates from whole grains, fruits, and vegetables. Emphasize the need for moderation and balance in carbohydrate intake, particularly for those with specific dietary requirements or goals.

Fat Phobia:

* ❖ **Challenge:** The misconception that all dietary fats are unhealthy and should be avoided can lead to inadequate intake of essential fatty acids and fat-soluble vitamins.
* ❖ **Addressing the misconception:** Educate individuals about the different types of fats, emphasizing the importance of consuming sources of healthy fats such as avocados, nuts, seeds, and olive oil. Encourage moderation and balance in fat consumption while avoiding sources of unhealthy fats like trans fats.

Lack of Nutrition Knowledge:

* ❖ **Challenge:** Many people lack basic nutrition knowledge, leading to confusion about what constitutes a healthy diet and making informed food choices.
* ❖ **Addressing the challenge:** Provide accessible and evidence-based nutrition education. Share reliable resources, encourage individuals to consult registered dietitians or nutritionists for personalized guidance, and emphasize the importance of staying informed about current nutrition research.

Emotional Eating and Food Guilt:

- ❖ **Challenge:** Emotional eating and feelings of guilt associated with food choices can negatively impact overall well-being and hinder progress towards fitness goals.
- ❖ **Addressing the challenge:** Promote mindful eating practices, self-compassion, and a non-restrictive approach to food. Encourage individuals to listen to their bodies, honor their hunger and fullness cues, and develop a healthy relationship with food that includes enjoyment and moderation.

By addressing these challenges and misconceptions, individuals can develop a more balanced and sustainable approach to nutrition, supporting their overall health and fitness goals. Providing accurate information and promoting a positive mindset around food can help individuals make informed choices and cultivate a healthy relationship with nutrition.

CHAPTER FOUR: STRENGTH TRAINING

THE BENEFITS OF STRENGTH TRAINING FOR

Strength training, also known as resistance training or weightlifting, offers numerous benefits for overall fitness and well-being. Here are some key benefits of incorporating strength training into your fitness routine:

- ❖ **Overall fitness Increased Muscle Strength and Endurance:** Strength training involves resistance exercises that target specific muscle groups. Over time, this leads to increased muscle strength and endurance. Stronger muscles can enhance performance in various physical activities and daily tasks, such as lifting heavy objects, climbing stairs, or participating in sports.

- ❖ **Improved Body Composition:** Strength training can help improve body composition by increasing lean muscle mass and reducing body fat. Muscle tissue is more metabolically active than fat tissue, meaning that having a higher proportion of lean muscle can increase your resting metabolic rate, leading to more efficient calorie burning even at rest. This can be beneficial for weight management and achieving a leaner physique.

- ❖ **Enhanced Bone Health:** Regular strength training has a positive impact on bone health by increasing bone density and strength. It can help prevent or reduce the risk of osteoporosis, a condition characterized by weak and brittle bones. The stress placed on the bones during resistance exercises stimulates the formation of new bone tissue, promoting overall skeletal health.

- ❖ **Increased Metabolic Rate:** Strength training can boost your metabolism, leading to increased calorie expenditure even after your workout. This is known as the "afterburn effect" or excess post-exercise oxygen consumption (EPOC). The body requires more energy to repair and rebuild muscles after intense strength training sessions, which can result in additional calorie burn over time.

- ❖ **Enhanced Functional Strength and Stability:** Strength training improves functional strength, which is the ability to perform everyday activities with ease and efficiency. It enhances stability, balance, and coordination, reducing the risk of falls and injuries. Functional strength is particularly important as we age, helping to maintain independence and overall quality of life.

- ❖ **Improved Joint Health and Injury Prevention:** Strengthening the muscles around the joints can provide better support and stability, reducing the risk of joint injuries and improving joint health. Strength training exercises can help strengthen the muscles, tendons, and ligaments that support the joints, enhancing overall joint function and flexibility.
- ❖ **Boosted Mood and Mental Well-being:** Strength training has a positive impact on mental health and well-being. It stimulates the release of endorphins, the feel-good hormones that can elevate mood and reduce stress, anxiety, and symptoms of depression. Regular strength training can also improve self-confidence and body image, promoting a positive mindset.
- ❖ **Enhanced Athletic Performance:** Strength training is a key component of athletic training programs. It improves power, speed, agility, and overall athletic performance. Athletes in various sports, including runners, cyclists, swimmers, and team sports athletes, can benefit from incorporating strength training exercises specific to their sport.

Remember to consult with a qualified fitness professional or strength training coach to design a safe and effective strength training program tailored to your individual needs and goals. Gradually increase the intensity and challenge of your workouts over time to continue reaping the benefits of strength training.

While it's not possible to physically demonstrate exercises through text, I can provide you with a brief description and key points for proper form and technique for some key exercises. It's important to note that proper form is crucial for maximizing the benefits of exercises and minimizing the risk of injury. If you're new to strength training or unsure about proper form, it's recommended to seek guidance from a qualified fitness professional or trainer who can provide hands-on instruction. Here are descriptions of form and technique for a few common exercises:

Squats:

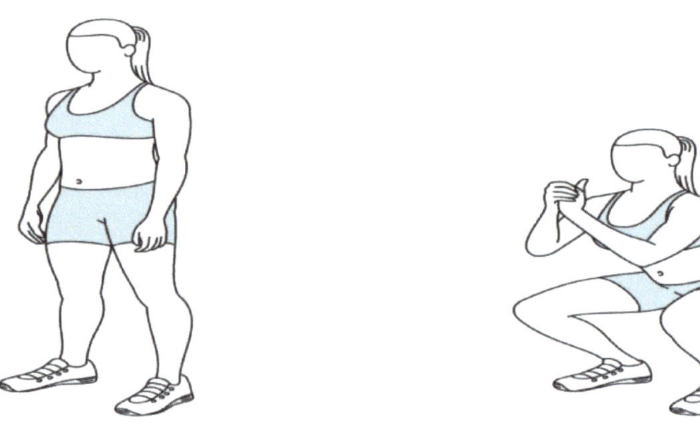

- ❖ Stand with your feet shoulder-width apart, toes pointing slightly outward.
- ❖ Engage your core, keep your chest lifted, and maintain a neutral spine throughout the movement.
- ❖ Bend your knees and lower your hips back and down, as if you're sitting into a chair.
- ❖ Lower until your thighs are parallel to the floor or slightly below, ensuring that your knees track over your toes.
- ❖ Push through your heels to return to the starting position, extending your hips and knees.

Push-Ups:

- ❖ Start in a high plank position with your hands slightly wider than shoulder-width apart, fingers pointing forward.
- ❖ Engage your core and maintain a straight line from your head to your heels.
- ❖ Lower your body by bending your elbows, keeping them at a 45-degree angle from your torso.
- ❖ Lower until your chest is just above the ground, then push through your palms to extend your arms and return to the starting position.

Deadlifts:

- ❖ Stand with your feet hip-width apart and the barbell centered over your feet.
- ❖ Hinge at your hips, maintaining a neutral spine, and grip the barbell with hands slightly wider than shoulder-width apart.
- ❖ Keep your chest lifted, engage your core, and press your shoulder blades down and back.
- ❖ Push through your heels, extend your hips and knees, and lift the barbell while maintaining a straight back.
- ❖ Reverse the movement by lowering the barbell back down, keeping it close to your body.

Dumbbell Shoulder Press:

- ❖ Start by holding dumbbells at shoulder level, palms facing forward, and elbows bent.
- ❖ Stand with your feet hip-width apart, engage your core, and maintain a neutral spine.
- ❖ Press the dumbbells overhead by extending your arms and fully straightening your elbows.
- ❖ Lower the dumbbells back down to shoulder level with control, maintaining stability and avoiding excessive arching of the back.

Remember, these descriptions provide a basic understanding of the exercises, but proper form and technique can vary based on individual needs, body mechanics, and equipment used. Always start with lighter weights to focus on mastering form before progressing to heavier loads. It's important to listen to your body, avoid any pain or discomfort, and modify exercises as needed. If possible, seek guidance from a qualified professional to ensure proper form and technique for your specific circumstances.

DEVELOPING A WELL-ROUNDED STRENGTH TRAINING PROGRAM

Developing a well-rounded strength training program involves targeting major muscle groups throughout the body to ensure balanced muscular development and functional strength. Here is a breakdown of the major muscle groups and exercises that target them:

Lower Body:

- ❖ **Quadriceps (front of the thighs):** Squats, lunges, leg press, leg extensions.
- ❖ **Hamstrings (back of the thighs):** Deadlifts, Romanian deadlifts, hamstring curls, glute bridges.
- ❖ **Glutes (buttocks):** Squats, hip thrusts, lunges, step-ups.
- ❖ **Calves:** Calf raises, standing calf raises.

Upper Body:

- ❖ **Chest**: Bench press, push-ups, dumbbell chest press, chest flyes.
- ❖ **Back:** Pull-ups, lat pulldowns, rows, deadlifts.
- ❖ **Shoulders:** Overhead press, lateral raises, front raises, upright rows.
- ❖ **Biceps:** Bicep curls, hammer curls, chin-ups.
- ❖ **Triceps:** Tricep dips, tricep pushdowns, overhead tricep extensions.

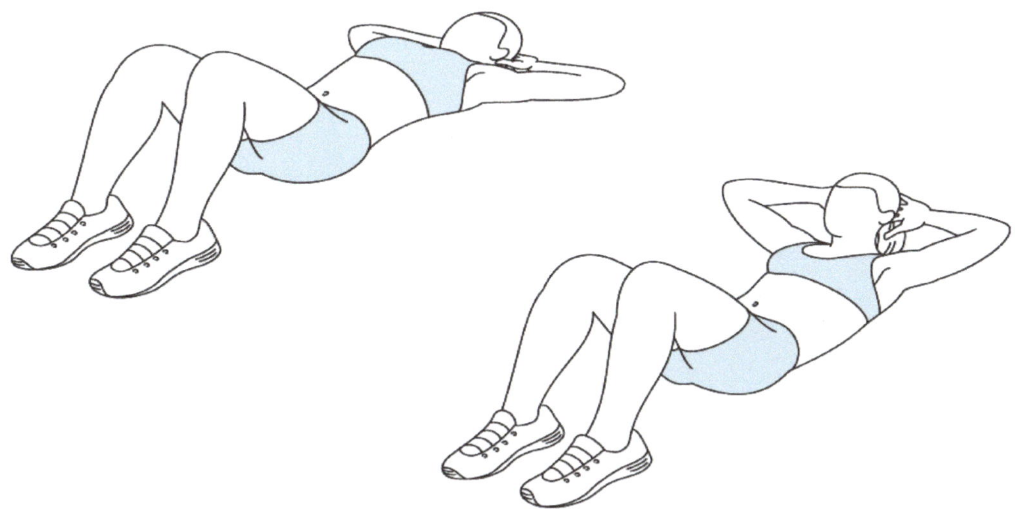

Core:

- **Rectus Abdominis (six-pack muscles):** Crunches, reverse crunches, planks.
- **Obliques (side abdominal muscles):** Russian twists, side planks, bicycle crunches.
- **Lower Back:** Superman, back extensions, hyperextensions.
- **Transverse Abdominis (deep core stability):** Dead bugs, bird dogs, plank variations.

Other Muscle Groups:

- **Deltoids (shoulder muscles):** Overhead press, lateral raises, front raises.
- **Trapezius (upper back and neck muscles):** Shrugs, upright rows.
- **Forearms:** Forearm curls, wrist curls, farmer's carries.
- **Lower Legs:** Tibialis anterior exercises (e.g., ankle dorsiflexion exercises) for shin muscles.

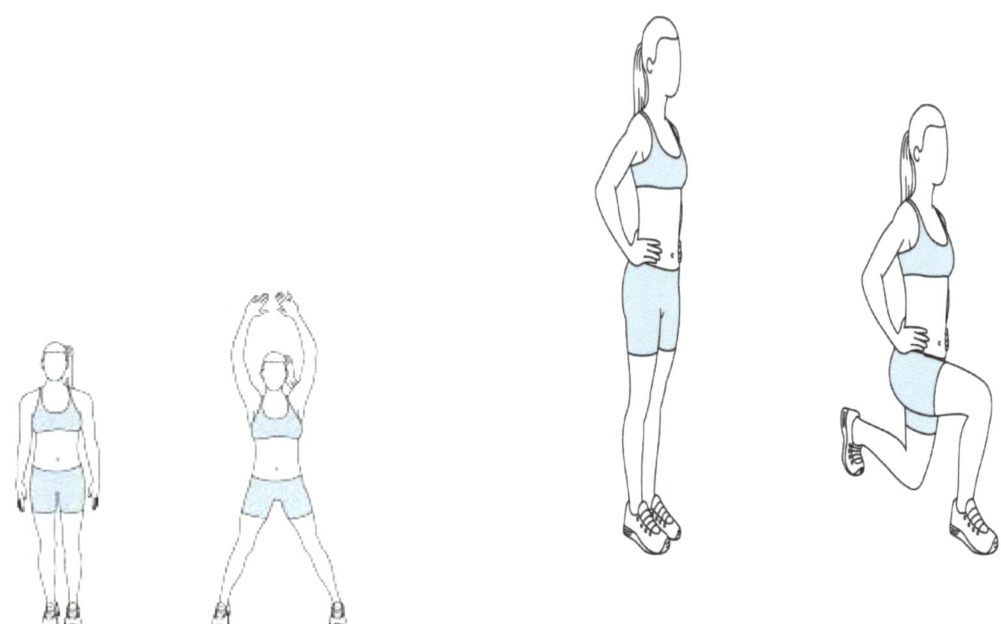

When designing your strength training program, aim for a balanced approach that includes exercises targeting each of these major muscle groups. Consider incorporating compound exercises that engage multiple muscle groups simultaneously, as well as isolation exercises that specifically target individual muscles.

Additionally, focus on using proper form and technique, gradually increasing resistance or difficulty, and allowing sufficient rest and recovery between sessions. It's also important to vary your exercises and incorporate different training modalities (e.g., free weights, bodyweight exercises, resistance bands) to challenge your muscles in different ways and prevent plateaus.

Remember to consult with a qualified fitness professional to tailor a strength training program to your specific goals, fitness level, and any individual considerations or limitations you may have. They can provide guidance on exercise selection, set and rep ranges, and progression strategies to help you achieve optimal results.

CHAPTER FIVE: RECOVERY AND INJURY PREVENTION

UNDERSTANDING THE IMPORTANCE OF RECOVERY FOR OPTIMAL FITNESS GAINS.

Understanding the importance of recovery is crucial for achieving optimal fitness gains. Here are some key points to highlight:

1. Muscular Repair and Growth: During exercise, muscles undergo stress and micro-tears. Adequate recovery allows the body to repair and rebuild these muscles, leading to increased strength and muscle growth. Without proper recovery, muscles may become overtrained, which can impede progress and increase the risk of injury.

2. Injury Prevention: Recovery plays a vital role in injury prevention. Rest periods allow the body to repair damaged tissues, reduce inflammation, and restore proper joint alignment. Failing to allow for sufficient recovery time can lead to overuse injuries and chronic pain.

3. Hormonal Balance: Intense exercise can disrupt hormonal balance, particularly the production of cortisol, commonly known as the stress hormone. Excessive cortisol levels can hinder muscle growth, impair immune function, and lead to fatigue and mood disturbances. Adequate recovery helps restore hormonal balance and promotes overall well-being.

4. Restoring Energy and Performance: Recovery allows for replenishment of energy stores, such as glycogen, in the muscles and liver. This replenishment enhances performance during subsequent workouts, enabling individuals to train at higher intensities and reach their fitness goals more effectively.

5. Mental and Emotional Well-being: Physical activity places demands not only on the body but also on the mind. Rest and recovery provide an opportunity to recharge mentally and emotionally. It can help reduce exercise-induced stress, improve mood, enhance concentration, and promote better sleep quality.

6. Adaptation and Progression: Recovery is essential for the body to adapt to the stresses imposed by exercise. It allows for the consolidation of strength gains, improvements in endurance, and other fitness adaptations. Consistently incorporating recovery periods into a training regimen helps individuals progress safely and sustainably over time.

7. Variety and Active Recovery: Recovery does not solely mean complete rest. Engaging in active recovery activities, such as light stretching, low-intensity exercises, or gentle movements, can enhance blood flow, aid in the removal of metabolic waste products, and reduce muscle soreness. Active recovery also provides a mental break from intense training while still promoting healing and recovery.

8. Sleep and Restful Breaks: Quality sleep is crucial for recovery. It is during sleep that the body repairs and regenerates tissues, balances hormone levels, and supports overall physical and mental health. Prioritizing regular, restful sleep helps optimize recovery and performance.

It's important to note that the ideal recovery strategy can vary based on factors such as individual goals, fitness level, and the intensity of training. However, incorporating rest days, active recovery, proper nutrition, adequate sleep, and stress management techniques are generally beneficial for optimizing recovery and achieving long-term fitness gains.

By understanding and prioritizing recovery as an integral part of your fitness journey, you can support your body's natural healing processes, reduce the risk of injury, and maximize the benefits of your training efforts.

EXPLORING VARIOUS RECOVERY TECHNIQUES: SLEEP, NUTRITION, ACTIVE REST, ETC

Exploring various recovery techniques is essential for promoting optimal fitness gains. Here are some effective recovery strategies to consider:

1. Quality Sleep: Adequate sleep is crucial for recovery. During sleep, the body undergoes processes that repair and rebuild tissues, regulate hormones, and support overall physical and mental well-being. Aim for 7-9 hours of quality sleep each night to facilitate optimal recovery.

2. Proper Nutrition: Fueling your body with nutritious foods is vital for recovery. Ensure you're consuming a balanced diet that includes a variety of whole foods, such as lean proteins, complex carbohydrates, healthy fats, and plenty of fruits and vegetables. Nutrient-dense meals and snacks provide the necessary building blocks for tissue repair and replenishment of energy stores.

3. Hydration: Proper hydration is essential for overall health and recovery. Drinking enough water helps maintain fluid balance, aids in nutrient transport, and supports optimal muscle function. Aim to drink water consistently throughout the day and adjust your intake based on activity level and environmental conditions.

4. Active Rest and Gentle Movement: Engaging in active rest days or incorporating gentle movement can aid in recovery. Light activities such as walking, yoga, or gentle stretching promote blood flow, increase nutrient delivery to muscles, and help alleviate muscle soreness. Active rest helps prevent stiffness and promotes a faster recovery without placing excessive stress on the body.

5. Foam Rolling and Self-Myofascial Release: Foam rolling and self-myofascial release techniques can help relieve muscle tension, improve flexibility, and enhance recovery. By applying gentle pressure to targeted areas, you can release knots, increase blood flow, and alleviate muscle soreness. Incorporate foam rolling into your routine, focusing on areas of tightness or discomfort.

6. Massage and Bodywork: Professional massage or other bodywork techniques can provide deep muscle relaxation, increase circulation, and promote recovery. Massage helps reduce muscle tension, improves range of motion, and enhances overall well-being. Consider scheduling regular massage sessions to support your recovery process.

7. Cold and Heat Therapy: Alternating between cold and heat therapy can aid in recovery. Cold therapy, such as ice baths or cold showers, helps reduce inflammation and muscle soreness. Heat therapy, such as hot baths or heating pads, promotes blood flow, relaxes muscles, and aids in recovery. Use these modalities as appropriate based on your individual needs and preferences.

8. Mindfulness and Stress Management: Incorporating mindfulness practices, such as meditation, deep breathing exercises, or relaxation techniques, can help reduce stress and promote recovery. Chronic stress can negatively impact recovery, so managing stress levels is crucial for optimal well-being.

9. Listen to Your Body: One of the most important recovery techniques is to listen to your body. Pay attention to signals of fatigue, soreness, or reduced performance. If needed, adjust your training intensity, duration, or frequency to allow for proper recovery. Remember that rest and recovery are just as important as training itself.

10. Periodization and Deloading: Incorporate planned periods of reduced training intensity or volume, known as deloading, into your program. Deloading allows for recovery, prevents overtraining, and promotes long-term progress. Periodization, which involves structured variations in training volume and intensity, also helps optimize recovery and performance.

It's important to note that recovery needs may vary based on individual factors such as fitness level, training intensity, and overall health. Experiment with different recovery techniques, listen to your body, and find what works best for you to support your overall well-being and fitness goals. Remember, recovery is a vital component of the training process and plays a key role in achieving long-term success.

PREVENTING COMMON EXERCISE-RELATED INJURIES THROUGH PROPER FORM AND TECHNIQUE.

Preventing exercise-related injuries is crucial for maintaining a safe and effective fitness routine. Here are some key points to highlight in terms of proper form and technique to minimize the risk of injuries:

1. Learn Proper Form: Before starting any exercise, take the time to learn and understand the correct form and technique. This may involve working with a qualified fitness professional, attending classes, or watching instructional videos. Proper form ensures that you engage the appropriate muscles and minimize unnecessary stress on joints and tissues.

2. Warm Up: Always start your workouts with a proper warm-up routine. This can include dynamic stretches, light cardio exercises, and mobility movements to prepare your muscles, joints, and cardiovascular system for the upcoming workout. Warming up increases blood flow, improves flexibility, and reduces the risk of injury.

3. Gradual Progression: Avoid the temptation to jump into high-intensity workouts or lift heavy weights before you have developed a solid foundation. Gradually increase the intensity, duration, and complexity of your exercises over time. This allows your body to adapt and strengthens the muscles, tendons, and ligaments necessary to support more challenging movements.

4. Focus on Core Stability: Develop a strong core to provide stability and support for your body during exercises. Engage your core muscles by drawing your belly button in toward your spine, maintaining proper alignment, and avoiding excessive arching or rounding of the back. Core stability helps prevent injuries and improves overall movement efficiency.

5. Listen to Your Body: Pay attention to any pain or discomfort during exercise. If you experience sharp or persistent pain, stop the exercise and consult with a healthcare professional. Pushing through pain can exacerbate an existing injury or lead to a new one. It's important to differentiate between muscle soreness, which is normal, and acute or chronic pain that requires attention.

6. Use Appropriate Equipment: Make sure you use the right equipment and gear for your workouts. This includes wearing proper athletic shoes with adequate support and cushioning, using appropriate weights and resistance bands, and ensuring equipment is in good working condition. Ill-fitting shoes or faulty equipment can increase the risk of injuries.

7. Modify as Needed: If you have any pre-existing conditions or limitations, modify exercises to suit your individual needs. This can involve reducing the range of motion, using lighter weights, or opting for alternative exercises that don't aggravate your condition. It's important to prioritize your safety and well-being during workouts.

8. Balance Strength and Flexibility: Maintain a balance between strength and flexibility training. Overly tight muscles can lead to imbalances and increased risk of injury, while excessive flexibility without adequate strength can also compromise stability. Incorporate stretching and mobility exercises into your routine to improve flexibility and maintain a balanced musculoskeletal system.

9. Recovery and Rest: Allow for proper recovery and rest days between workouts. Rest is essential for tissue repair and growth, and it helps prevent overuse injuries. Listen to your body's signals for fatigue and avoid pushing through excessive fatigue or pain.

10.   Seek Professional Guidance: If you're new to exercise or have specific concerns, consider working with a qualified fitness professional or physical therapist. They can provide personalized guidance, assess your movement patterns, and help you develop a safe and effective exercise program.

By prioritizing proper form, technique, and injury prevention strategies, you can significantly reduce the risk of exercise-related injuries. Remember to always listen to your body, make gradual progress, and prioritize your safety and well-being in your fitness journey.

REHABILITATION AND INJURY MANAGEMENT STRATEGIES.

Rehabilitation and injury management are crucial aspects of fitness to help individuals recover from injuries, regain strength, and safely return to their fitness routines. Here are some strategies to consider:

1. Seek Professional Evaluation: If you've experienced an injury, it's important to consult with a healthcare professional, such as a doctor, physical therapist, or sports medicine specialist. They can assess the severity of the injury, provide a diagnosis, and recommend appropriate treatment and rehabilitation strategies.

2. Follow the R.I.C.E. Principle: The R.I.C.E. principle stands for Rest, Ice, Compression, and Elevation. This approach is commonly used for acute injuries, such as sprains or strains. Rest the injured area, apply ice packs wrapped in a cloth to reduce swelling, use compression bandages to provide support, and elevate the injured limb above heart level to minimize swelling.

3. Adhere to Rehabilitation Protocols: Once you have a treatment plan from a healthcare professional, it's important to follow the prescribed rehabilitation protocols. This may involve specific exercises, stretches, or modalities such as heat or ultrasound therapy. Rehabilitation protocols are designed to promote healing, restore range of motion, and rebuild strength in the affected area.

4. Gradual Return to Activity: When recovering from an injury, it's essential to progress gradually back into your fitness routine. Start with low-impact exercises or modified versions of your usual activities, gradually increasing intensity and volume as tolerated. Listen to your body, and don't rush the recovery process to avoid reinjury.

5. Focus on Functional Movements: Incorporate exercises that improve functional movements and help restore normal movement patterns. This can include exercises that promote balance, stability, coordination, and proprioception. Working with a physical therapist or qualified fitness professional can help guide you in selecting appropriate exercises for your specific injury.

6. Strengthen the Supporting Muscles: In many cases, injury can lead to muscle imbalances or weakness in surrounding areas. It's important to address these imbalances through targeted strength training. Focus on strengthening the supporting muscles around the injured area to promote stability and prevent future injuries.

7. Modify Activities as Needed: During the recovery process, you may need to modify certain activities or exercises to accommodate your injury. This may involve using lighter weights, reducing range of motion, or opting for alternative exercises that don't put excessive strain on the injured area. Work with a professional to develop modified exercises that allow you to continue training safely.

8. Incorporate Cross-Training: Cross-training involves engaging in different types of exercises or activities to reduce the strain on specific muscle groups or joints. Incorporating low-impact activities such as swimming, cycling, or using an elliptical machine can help maintain cardiovascular fitness while minimizing stress on the injured area.

9. Focus on Flexibility and Mobility: Injury can lead to stiffness and decreased range of motion. Incorporate stretching and mobility exercises to improve flexibility, enhance joint mobility, and prevent further restrictions in movement. Pay attention to stretching both the injured area and surrounding muscles to maintain overall flexibility.

10. Patience and Mental Resilience: Rehabilitation can be a challenging and time-consuming process. It's important to maintain a positive mindset, be patient with the recovery timeline, and stay committed to the rehabilitation program. Building mental resilience and seeking support from healthcare professionals or support groups can help you navigate the emotional aspects of injury recovery.

Remember, rehabilitation and injury management should always be guided by healthcare professionals who can provide personalized advice based on your specific injury and circumstances. Following proper rehabilitation protocols, gradually returning to activity, and prioritizing injury prevention strategies can help you recover safely and get back to your fitness routine.

STRATEGIES FOR AVOIDING OVERTRAINING AND BURNOUT.

Avoiding overtraining and burnout is crucial for maintaining long-term health, preventing injuries, and sustaining motivation in your fitness journey. Here are some strategies to consider:

1. Listen to Your Body: Pay attention to your body's signals and respond accordingly. If you're feeling excessively fatigued, experiencing persistent muscle soreness, or noticing a decline in performance, it may be a sign of overtraining. Take rest days or reduce the intensity and volume of your workouts when needed.

2. Plan Adequate Recovery: Allow for proper recovery between workouts. This includes incorporating rest days into your training schedule and prioritizing sleep and relaxation. Recovery is essential for muscle repair, hormone balance, and overall well-being. Aim for 1-2 rest days per week and prioritize quality sleep of 7-9 hours each night.

3. Vary Your Training: Incorporate variety into your training routine. This can involve changing exercise modalities, trying new activities, or exploring different training methods. Varying your workouts not only helps prevent overuse injuries but also keeps your routine interesting and enjoyable.

4. Practice Periodization: Utilize the concept of periodization, which involves systematically varying training intensity and volume over specific periods. This allows for adequate recovery and adaptation, reducing the risk of overtraining. Include planned deload weeks or mesocycles with lower intensity to promote recovery and prevent burnout.

5. Set Realistic Goals: Set goals that are challenging yet attainable. Unrealistic goals or a constant focus on pushing your limits can lead to excessive stress and burnout. Break down your goals into smaller milestones and celebrate achievements along the way to maintain motivation and prevent feeling overwhelmed.

6. Incorporate Active Recovery: Include active recovery days or lighter workouts into your routine. Engaging in low-intensity activities such as yoga, gentle stretching, or light cardio can help promote blood flow, reduce muscle soreness, and provide a mental break from intense training.

7. Prioritize Self-Care: Take time for self-care activities that help you relax and recharge. This can include activities like meditation, mindfulness exercises, taking walks in nature, engaging in hobbies, or spending quality time with loved ones. Prioritizing self-care helps manage stress levels and prevent burnout.

8. Manage Stress: Identify and manage sources of stress in your life. Chronic stress can contribute to overtraining and burnout. Implement stress management techniques such as deep breathing exercises, journaling, or engaging in activities that help you unwind and reduce stress levels.

9. Seek Support: Surround yourself with a supportive community of like-minded individuals who can provide encouragement, accountability, and guidance. Consider working with a fitness coach

or joining fitness classes where instructors can help structure your training and provide guidance on proper progression.

10.	Enjoy the Process: Remember to find joy in your fitness journey. Focus on the process rather than solely fixating on outcomes. Celebrate small victories, appreciate the improvements in strength or endurance, and maintain a positive mindset. Enjoying the process makes it more sustainable and reduces the likelihood of burnout.

It's important to remember that everyone's training capacity and recovery needs are unique. Pay attention to your individual circumstances, adjust your training accordingly, and always prioritize your well-being. By implementing these strategies, you can reduce the risk of overtraining and burnout, allowing for consistent progress and long-term fitness success.

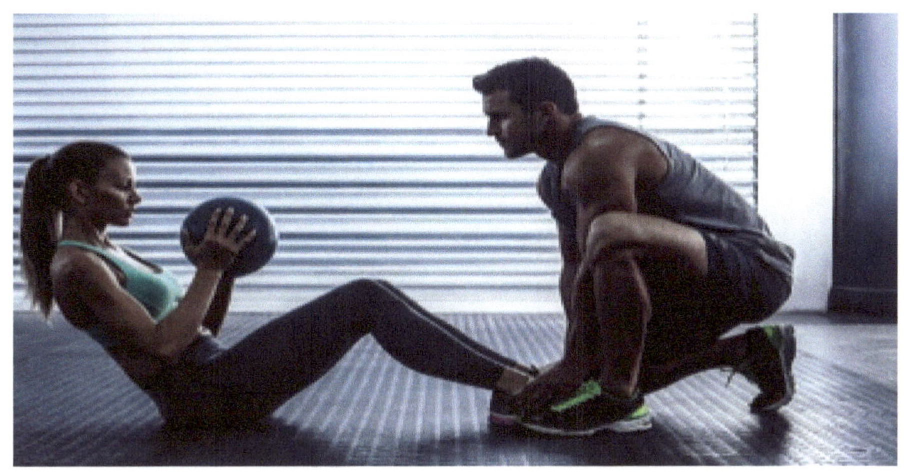

CONCLUSION:

In conclusion, this book provides readers with a comprehensive guide to achieving and maintaining optimal fitness. It emphasizes the importance of adopting a holistic approach to fitness, encompassing physical, mental, and emotional well-being. The book covers various components of fitness, including cardiovascular endurance, muscular strength and endurance, flexibility, and body composition. It explores the benefits of regular exercise and physical activity, debunks common fitness myths, and provides strategies for assessing individual fitness levels and setting SMART goals.

The book delves into the role of nutrition in achieving fitness goals, discussing macronutrients, micronutrients, and strategies for balanced and healthy eating. It highlights the significance of strength training and provides guidance on proper form, technique, and designing personalized strength training programs. It also explores the importance of cardiovascular exercise, different types of cardio activities, and creating effective cardio workout routines.

The book addresses the importance of flexibility and mobility, introducing stretching techniques, mobility exercises, and foam rolling. It discusses the connection between mental well-being and physical fitness, explores mindfulness, meditation, and stress management techniques, and incorporates yoga and Pilates for improved flexibility, strength, and mental clarity.

Furthermore, the book provides strategies for maintaining motivation, overcoming setbacks, and fostering a positive mindset. It emphasizes the importance of recovery, explores various recovery techniques, and provides guidance on preventing injuries and managing rehabilitation. Additionally, it addresses the importance of seeking professional guidance and support from trainers, coaches, and fitness communities.

Overall, this book aims to empower readers with the knowledge and tools to create a personalized fitness plan, overcome obstacles, and achieve long-term success in their fitness journey. By implementing the principles and strategies outlined in this book, readers can transform their lives, improve their physical fitness, and enhance their overall well-being.